For Kok Fai Soong, my father, with love.

The goldfish in the garden pond miss you, and so do I. Rest in peace.

Contents

Why Pharmacy?

So, why Pharmacy? Did you fail medical school interviews?

If I'm being honest, my decision to study Pharmacy was a fairly unremarkable one. There was no eureka moment. There was no dramatic parting of the clouds, and there was most certainly no choir of angels singing from on high.

I'd be lying if I told you I was fulfilling a lifelong passion and burning desire to become a legal drug aficionado. I enjoyed chemistry, I was curious about the science of drug development, and I had somehow achieved the right grades for the right A-levels. That was that. Off I went to dedicate the next five years of my life to the pursuit of Pharmacy in the big city.

In fact, I nearly became a concert violinist. But that's a story for another day.

The first day of university arrived. Feeling like a lost sheep who had wandered too far from home for the first time (I mean this very literally - I walked into the wrong lecture theatre many a time), I was a frazzled ball of nerves disguised as a wide-eyed fresher. I was as fresh as freshers get. Fresh from the crisp air of the Somerset countryside to the streets of London, where phone-snatching criminals on mopeds are drawn to unsuspecting individuals with phones in hand like flies to honey. I could not have felt more out of place.

Only ten per cent of you will graduate with first class honours, they said. Some of you won't make it past the first year at all. By the end of day one, I had concluded that I knew absolutely nothing about Pharmacy.

Over the next few years, I would come to realise how right I was. I had no idea what a pharmacist did, or was capable of. I even dropped the condescending "pill counting" quip a fair few times myself. Nevertheless, I would eventually learn that there was so much more to the world of pharmacy and pharmaceutical science – and just how ignorant I had been. I would eventually see for myself the complexities of decision making in healthcare, and how the most truthful answer to a patient's question is often "I don't know". Eventually, I would fall in love with the art of pharmaceutical formulation and drug delivery. So much so that I was willing to add a year to the sufficiently arduous

MPharm degree to venture into the pharmaceutical industry and experience it for myself.

This book is a compilation of my experiences in pharmacy, as well as some thoughts on healthcare and the pharmaceutical industry. If you are considering a Pharmacy degree, I hope this little project of mine can give you an insight into the journey that lies ahead of you – or at least the start of it. It is so much more than coursework deadlines, all-nighters and mountains of textbooks. It is most definitely a whole lot more than pill counting.

If you are a qualified pharmacist and have been practising for a while now, maybe you'll get a few giggles out of my bumbling student misfortunes, or at least enjoy a little nostalgia for the good old days of pharmacy school. Most of all, whether you work in pharmacy or not, I hope it makes you smile a little. And maybe think a little.

To answer the question at the start of this chapter, the answer is no - I did not fail medical school interviews. I never applied.

I don't think the medical world is ready for my idea of bedside manner that involves telling a patient that their COPD[1] diagnosis is their fault for decades of chain-smoking, and they need to get their shit

---

[1] COPD – Chronic obstructive pulmonary disease

together. Honestly, I don't think I'd make it to the "I want to save lives" part of the interview.

Legal Drug Dealer on Speed (Dial)

As soon as your Pharmacy student credentials crop up in conversation, people tend to respond in one of several ways; the most common being the legal drug dealer joke. If I had a penny for the number of times I've had to fake-laugh at this, I'd be a millionaire by now. Student loans? Ha, what are those?

When the legal drug dealer joke has been milked dry, Breaking Bad references and Walter White comparisons usually follow, along with the usual suggestions of making meth and becoming an internationally renowned crime lord.

Given the right equipment, I could probably – very hypothetically speaking – make you your very own batch of crystal meth. Though I think the GPhC[2] might be less supportive of my crime lord aspirations.

---

[2] GPhC – General Pharmaceutical Council. The independent regulator for pharmacists and pharmacy technicians in the United Kingdom.

Alternatively, you may get the classic "Oh, you're a pharmacist?" and the eyes of the opportunists around you will light up like fireflies in a marsh. No matter how fervently you shake your head in denial at this point and reiterate that you are still in training, there isn't much you can do to prevent the ensuing onslaught of healthcare-themed questions. Think stampede, à la The Lion King. You may get a few enthusiastic offers from family and friends (or strangers) to show you their lumps and bumps. Sometimes, it might be a rash located on a body part that conveniently requires them to strip. If you're lucky, you may even get a case of athlete's foot thrust in your face for your appraisal.

Once in a blue moon, you may get other kinds of comments. You may be asked why you didn't just do medicine instead. Doctors are more important and make more money, don't they? Do you want to stand behind a counter for the rest of your life?

That last one has to be my personal favourite.

I think these folks deserve a whole chapter of their own. I will thus leave them for now and ask you kindly to put them at the back of your mind as you work your way through the book. Always leave your audience wanting more – at least that's what I've been told.

Or you could just turn to Chapter 20. Patience is a virtue, but it certainly isn't one of mine.

Nonetheless, I conclude this chapter with a little anecdote from a friend. I wish I could say I had the pleasure of witnessing this encounter, but this regrettably only reached me through the gossip vine. Just know that I would give anything to have been a fly on the wall that night – just about anything.

In my first year of university, I had a friend who enjoyed the London clubbing scene, something commonly and fondly associated with being in your early twenties and being a fresher. She was a regular at the usual favourite spots amongst students – multiple times a week, to be exact. One fateful night, she caught the eye of a certain someone across the dance floor. As soon as their eyes met, the electricity was palpable. The air between them shimmered with tension, and time seemed to stand still.

I am not a clubber. Could you tell?

After what I assume was some intense eye-humping (for want of a better description), they eventually got to small talk over an overpriced drink or two. Everything seemed to be going well until she told him that she was studying to become a pharmacist.

7

"Oh, you need a degree for that?"

Suffice to say, they never saw each other again.

Never Stop Learning

I've started to notice a pattern when it comes to navigating this healthcare thing. Just as I start to think I've reached a level where I stand a chance of being slightly useful in a clinical environment, something or someone always comes along to remind me just how little I actually know. They weren't kidding when they said you never stop learning.

Let's put it this way – over the years, I've learned to get comfortable with being the clueless one in the room.

I used to think that nystatin was a statin. Prior to finding out that this was not the case, I had devised a revision shortcut that I was rather proud of and if I might say so myself, it had been pretty successful - until then. To help me mentally compartmentalise drugs within their respective classes for efficient learning, I'd noticed that drugs of a similar class tend to share the same suffix. Drugs of a suffix flock together, if you will. For example, beta blockers end in "-olol" – take bisoprolol, atenolol or propranolol. Penicillins end in "-cillin" –

phenoxymethylpenicillin, flucloxacillin, or amoxicillin (I hear the banana flavoured stuff tastes great). It might therefore not come as much of a surprise that statins end in "-statin". Atorvastatin, simvastatin – bonus points for creativity, really.

Imagine my shock when I came across nystatin. Finding out that it was (still is) an antifungal and not a statin had thrown a wrench into my little system that had been running like clockwork so far. Were there other exceptions in other drug classes? How many were there? How dare these impostors crash my party and turn it into a damn drug masquerade?

Once you've figured out which drug belongs to which class, trying to pronounce them correctly opens up a whole new bonus level of the game - "trying" being the keyword. You see, being able to say them in my head or mumble them under my breath is not enough. One day, I'll find myself sitting down with a patient to have a conversation about their new medication – as their pharmacist. They'll smile outwardly, but also somehow simultaneously make eye contact with me and the nearest clock, as if to communicate how precious their time is and I'd better have something ground-breaking to tell them about this drug. Or at the very least, be able to pronounce it correctly.

God forbid, they'll learn from my pronunciation and tell people, "That's how the pharmacist said it". There's no turning back after that. I don't think the old quick mumbling trick will cut it this time.

In my deepest, darkest fantasies, getting through a whole conversation about a drug without having to utter its name once is perfectly acceptable. In these fantasies, I am also a billionaire in a world where unicorns exist and dogs talk.

I've heard all sort of colourful pronunciations from patients, peers and pharmacists alike. Even in my limited number of years in Pharmacy to date, I have learned that the line between the "correct" pronunciation and "everything else" is often blurred to the point of non-existence. I've heard "settee-zyne" for cetirizine. "Preggy-ball" for pregabalin. "Brufen" for ibuprofen.

Ironically, Brufen does in fact exist – as a proprietary name for ibuprofen. Mylan (well, Abbott) clearly knew what they were doing.

That's just to name a few. I have to hand it to these people; I don't think I could make up better ones if I tried. When I include a line in my CV describing my experience in "handling patient requests for repeat prescriptions", rest assured that I really mean "playing a game of guess-the-drug". Sometimes, patients even threw me a curveball to check if I was still awake – "please could I have more of the round white tablets?"

I hate to break it to you, but most of them are round and white. Trust me, it inconveniences me just as much as it does you.

Riddle me this, though. Abciximab. Ab-*six*-imab? Or ab-*kick*-simab?

I think I'd rather be kicked in the abs at this point.

Eau de Salbutamol

There are certain people you just don't forget. They waltz into your life and make their mark on you with a certain *je ne sais quoi*, and you find yourself wondering about them every so often. Before you know it, they've carved out a spot for themselves on your "unforgettable people" list.

I used to work Saturdays as a counter assistant in a local pharmacy. This weekend gig killed two birds with one stone – I became much more familiar with the ins and outs of retail pharmacy, and pocket money trickled steadily into my bank account each month. A particularly delightful patient I met during a shift at the pharmacy proved herself more than worthy of my "unforgettable people" list the day I met her. We'll call her Barbara.

Barbara was an elderly lady who called everyone "dear" and always had a kind smile to spare – the type that hypnotises you into smiling right back before you realise what your cheek muscles are doing. She had a question for the pharmacist that day. As the pharmacist was busy

13

with another patient, I apologised and offered her a chair whilst she waited. I then asked if there was anything else I could assist her with in the meantime.

"Well, you see dear – these inhalers just don't work!"

Barbara was asthmatic and her doctor had prescribed her these nifty little pieces of technology that, she was told, would help with her shortness of breath. She told me that she had been using her inhaler exactly as she had been instructed. She said she was doing the required two puffs twice a day. Yet she insisted that she had seen no improvement in her symptoms. Maybe these just aren't for me, she said. I then asked her if she could show me how she was using the inhalers.

Taking the cap off her inhaler, she spritzed either side of her neck – two puffs, just as she had told me. For good measure, she wafted the mist about with her hand and inhaled.

I did eventually manage to pick my jaw up off the floor. Inhalers can be tricky. I'll be honest – I have never used one myself, simply from lack of need. I've been taught to counsel patients to "inhale fast and deep" for a dry powder inhaler, or "inhale slow and deep" for a pressured metered-dose inhaler. I also know that I should remind them to exhale fully before using the inhaler, and to hold their breath for ten seconds after inhaling. Other than that, I'm just as much at the mercy of that origami-esque patient information leaflet as you are.

Barbara – wherever you are– one of these days, someone might just develop inhaled bronchodilator therapy that smells so good they call it Barbara No. 5. Now that's a world I want to live in.

When Antibiotics Crashed the Warfarin Party

Interprofessional education workshops. Ah, it's that time of year again. That time of year when students from a multitude of healthcare professions get together from far and wide. Bright-eyed and bushy-tailed, they frolic with joyous abandon in the myriad of mysteries also known as simulated patient cases.

No matter how much students complain about having to attend these sessions, everyone almost always leaves pleasantly surprised at how much fun they had. We don't get to meet students from other disciplines often, yet we are somehow expected to fully understand everyone's unique skillsets in the workplace immediately after graduation. Interprofessional education workshops present a great opportunity for us to take responsibility for the care of mock patients as an interdisciplinary team.

It's a little like playing a pharmacist in the Sims games. In these sessions, "Patient X" may be no more than a description on paper, but

16

he looks to us for answers. And we're damn well expected to find them. Or at least start by figuring out how to work together.

I had been assigned to the case of Patient MK, along with three medics and two nursing students. Patient MK was an elderly lady who had been admitted to a busy hospital ward with a chest infection and she had been prescribed some antibiotics for this. To make matters more interesting, she was also taking warfarin due to a recent mitral valve replacement[3].

Warfarin is an anticoagulant that "thins" the blood and reduces the chances of the patient's blood clotting. When blood clots form and travel around the body, they turn into little ticking time bombs. Once they get to the heart or brain, shit goes down.

By shit, I mean a stroke or a myocardial infarction, where the clot blocks blood flow and cells start to die suddenly due to lack of oxygen. Needless to say, anticoagulation is a huge priority in the care of patients who may be more predisposed to clotting – i.e. patients who have had a valve replacement. This immediately puts Patient MK in the red danger zone.

---

[3] A mitral valve replacement is an operation where the mitral valve in the heart is replaced with a mechanical or bioprosthetic valve.

Warfarin is also a high-maintenance drug, much like a needy dog that needs to be checked on every so often to keep it out of trouble. This happens in the form of regular INR monitoring, a standard requirement for every patient started on warfarin. INR stands for "international normalised ratio". In a nutshell, it represents the time taken for a patient's blood to clot, thus helping clinicians determine the best dose of warfarin for an individual. Too much warfarin and the patient's INR shoots up; the longer it takes for their blood to clot, the higher their risk of bleeding. Too little warfarin and their INR is too low – anticoagulation is inadequate and they are still at risk of a stroke or myocardial infarction. For a prosthetic mitral valve replacement, we're looking at a target INR of 2-3[10].

The pharmacist in this scenario then uncovers that Patient MK hasn't had her INR checked since admission, and requests that this be done immediately. Following a series of miscommunications and what I like to call "responsibility ping-pong" amongst the ward staff, Patient MK's INR never gets checked and a nurse gives her a dose of warfarin that evening as per usual.

The next morning, MK suffers not one, but two severe nose bleeds. It somehow takes the Niagara Falls of nosebleeds to spur these fictional healthcare professionals into action. They finally check her INR and it turns out to be a whopping 7.4. We've gone to infinity and way beyond our target of 2-3.

Now, why did the nose bleeds happen? After getting past the incompetence of the ward staff in this story, we got to unwrapping the core of the problem. It was decided that Patient MK's bleeding was most likely due to warfarin overexposure. But how did this happen? As far as the story goes, she had been taking it as per usual. There was no intentional or accidental overdosing that we know of. Nothing was out of the ordinary.

Except for the antibiotics.

I piped up, suggesting that the antibiotics may have caused the warfarin overexposure. Certain antibiotics can increase warfarin levels in the blood by inhibiting the breakdown of warfarin, so that there is more warfarin available in the body for longer. Therefore, more warfarin equals an increase in the patient's INR, putting them at a higher risk of bleeding even when the patient has been taking the same dose of warfarin as they always have been.

I was met with five blank faces.

"Really? Antibiotics can do that?" Whilst I was bombarded with questions left, right and centre, my ego swelled in a majestic crescendo. Which antibiotics interact with warfarin? Does this happen with any other drugs, and how on earth did I know this? I proceeded to tell them about the principles of enzyme inhibition and induction and how this relates to drug metabolism. I had naively assumed that all healthcare disciplines would know this and I would simply be stating the obvious by exposing Patient MK's new antibiotics as a key suspect. Boy was I wrong.

I guess you do learn a thing or two in Pharmacy after all.

Just Keep Running

Like many hopeful runners-to-be, I woke up one day and decided it was time I tried the Couch-to-5k programme. As the name suggests, Couch-to-5k is an app that aims to get you running a full five kilometres, no matter your current level of fitness or experience. It provides a structured training plan designed to whip you into a decent enough shape to achieve your 5k goal in an ambitious nine weeks.

Herein lies my greatest obstacle – I am a much bigger fan of the couch than I am of running continuously for half an hour. The couch envelops me in its forgiving folds and lovingly cushions my own folds. It doesn't tear my self-esteem down every time an uphill stretch leaves me winded. It doesn't make my lungs burn and serve as an ever-present reminder of how much my legs will ache the next day, as I pound the pavement in an attempt to get fit.

Pharmacists are expected to promote a healthy lifestyle. We are taught to recommend at least one hundred and fifty minutes of moderate-intensity activity a week for an average adult[13]. We are told to recommend a balanced diet, offer you smoking cessation services, and tell you that you shouldn't drink more than fourteen units of alcohol a week.

We (at least some of us) also don't always practise what we preach.

During my time as a counter assistant in that local pharmacy down the road, I often found myself rattling off these healthcare mantras to customers and patients. Drink enough fluids, prioritise exercise, get enough sleep – the list goes on. In fact, my brain was often busy concocting a new flavour combination for my next no-bake cheesecake – whilst these pieces of advice were coming out of my mouth on autopilot.

Raspberry cheesecake with a chocolate biscuit base, anyone?

At the end of the day, I would go home and sit down for the rest of the evening and of course, the couch would welcome me with open arms. I felt like a hypocrite for not doing these things I was promoting so enthusiastically to others without thinking twice. So, I took my own advice and started running.

Enter the Couch-to-5k programme. The training plan is designed for beginners – the level zeros of the running world, if you will. It sets reasonable, achievable goals from week to week that slowly but surely, take you from walking most of the thirty-minute session to running it in its entirety by week nine. Best of all, it's free. Big tick for the happy student box.

Week one was surprisingly manageable. One minute of running followed by one and a half minutes of walking – this wasn't so bad. What a confidence booster. I completed week one fuelled by my "Cheesy Eighties Hits" playlist, feeling on top of the world. I was ready to become a runner.

However, each week got progressively more difficult, and I started to hit a wall around week four. Three to five minutes of continuous running had me wheezing like an asthmatic horse, whilst runners more than twice my age lapped me multiple times along my running route. By the time I reached week seven, hay fever season had started. Whilst the flowers bloomed and the bees and the butterflies flitted about without a care in the world, I became familiar with the art of sneeze-running, accompanied by bouts of enthusiastic snot wiping.

Thank modern science for antihistamines.

Eventually, I completed the program. I had finally graduated from the couch to running five kilometres three times a week. Those nine weeks were a steep uphill climb – mentally, physically and literally. I sweated from crevices I didn't know I could sweat from. There were times where I had somehow left the steepest uphill sections of my route for the end of the run, and my legs were crying out for me to stop. There were times when I had to slow to a walk mid-run, just so that I could complete the whole session. There were runs that I could not complete at all.

I will never again judge an overweight patient who struggles with the "lifestyle advice" part of the consultation. Life is much simpler when you can just pop a statin and be done with it.

Here's an even bigger miracle for you - I still run five kilometres three times a week. Truth be told, I'm a slow runner – it's the only way I can get through the entirety of the run without stopping. My average pace probably clocks in at the lower end of a car in first gear. I do all the running motions fairly convincingly, but I'm pretty sure I only ever move at walking speed.

Maybe I should be an illusionist next. I can hear my couch telling me to go for it.

Sense and Sensibility in Death and Disability

I lost Dad to terminal cancer not too long ago. Lung cancer with brain metastases and leptomeningeal disease.

That changed the mood quickly, didn't it?

I remember the day I received word of the diagnosis. It came in the form of a cheerful ding, alerting me to an unassuming email notification on my phone. I remember being frozen to the spot as I read it over and over, desperately hoping I had misread it the first time. I also remember crying as I have never cried before. Barely able to see through my tears, I frantically googled the prognosis of stage IV non-small-cell lung cancer.

For a patient diagnosed at such an advanced stage of disease, the five-year survival rate tends to be less than ten percent.

Five years, ten percent. No - less than ten percent.

25

No matter how many sources I consulted, they all told me the same thing. I went through all the journal articles and webpages I could find on the subject. I convinced myself that I had at least five years left with him – and desperately tried to ignore how unrealistic and optimistic this was.

Two years later, we were told that the targeted therapy – that had been so successful until then – was ceasing to control tumour growth. Don't worry, we have options - they said. The next drug turned out to be just as ineffective. Don't worry, we have more options - they said. Then they discovered the brain metastases.

Guess what? They had options. But this was *the* warning. The warning that we should begin to prepare ourselves.

The ticking clock of reality had reared its ugly head one last time.

Despite the chemotherapy sessions and the many survival statistics we were fed in an attempt to give us hope, nothing seemed to work. As the secondary brain tumour had spread to the meninges[4], surgery was not an option. Dad began to decline at an alarming rate. Before we knew it, we found ourselves sitting by his bed in the hospice. His room

---

[4] Meninges – the three protective layers of thin membrane that surround the brain and spinal cord.

overlooked a koi pond and a sprawling garden with vegetables and herbs of every kind. It could not have been more perfect for him. We played his favourite music whilst he spent more and more of every day asleep.

It was 20 July 2019. The sun shone and we had just spotted a heron by the pond. Dad had finally slipped into the most peaceful sleep of his life.

Somehow, I thought that my training to become a healthcare professional would give me the emotional tools I needed to deal with this. I assumed I would be more prepared for the day I would lose him. In truth, I had already lost him to the disease a while before he passed – the combination of the aggressive malignancy and the daily cocktail of drugs had left him a shell of his former self. I convinced myself that I would be ready when the moment came. I foolishly thought that maintaining an intellectual perspective on his disease management would be enough to distract me from the emotional hurricane that threatened to wreak havoc on my self-composure at any moment. Maybe I could apply the same objective clarity to this situation as I had been trained to do with any other patient.

But he wasn't any other patient. There was nothing I could have done to prepare myself.

I was foolish to think that I could have convinced myself otherwise. I was far from prepared – for the moment he passed or for the many other moments of unbridled pain that I would continue to experience afterwards. A few months on, I was in a lecture theatre taking notes on how some injections had to be formulated as an acidic preparation for the sake of preserving drug stability, but could be painful for the patient on injection. Before I knew it, all I could think about was Dad's pained gasps as the hospice nurse gave him his daily corticosteroid injections. We learned about the benefits and limitations of new pharmacological developments in oncology. I was so painfully familiar with the names of these drugs that I recorded them in my notes as two-letter abbreviations, whilst everyone else joked that pharma companies just wanted to make these names as difficult to pronounce as possible.

They don't tell us much about these things at university. There are no lectures on how to approach the subject of mortality with a patient and their family. We don't get taught much about handling disability in practice either.

Maybe these topics are explored on a deeper level within other healthcare disciplines where graduates are more likely to encounter them than your average pharmacist. However, I can confidently say that no amount of training in handling "sensitive topics" could have prepared me for losing Dad. It almost seems coldly arrogant to think that I could have been ready at all.

I also have one request for the healthcare professionals amongst you.

For the first time, I understood a patient's desperation. I understood what it meant to be willing to do anything – anything at all – just to buy a little bit more time with a loved one. My mother and I spent sleepless nights researching new therapies available and scoured the web for relevant clinical trials featuring experimental drugs in advanced non-small cell lung cancer. As someone who has undertaken formal training in healthcare, it can be easy to scoff at patients and families who do this. It is easy to brush them off with a condescending smile and an apologetic "no" – do they really think their home "research" stands a chance against years of rigorous professional training?

Not a single member of Dad's oncology team did this. They accepted our findings with genuine interest, and answered all our questions with a degree of patience and honesty that was second to none. There wasn't a single patronising smile in sight.

I didn't realise it at the time, but this is the core of patient-centred care. This is what it's all about.

So, the next time Mrs. Jones walks into your pharmacy screeching about her blood pressure pills for the tenth time that week, suppress the urge to roll your eyes. Sometimes, her underlying concerns may be much, much bigger than the issue of why she hasn't received this month's Amlodipine supply yet. And that is where the real challenge lies.

Money Makes the World Go Round

You've probably seen the tabloid headlines branding pharmaceutical companies as money-grabbing snakes. Martin Shkreli and his pyrimethamine exploits certainly didn't discourage this image. Whilst the NHS[5] keeps prescription charges at a minimum (albeit a slowly climbing one) in the UK, people subject to healthcare systems elsewhere may not be as lucky. If you talk to any patient whose quality of life has been at the mercy of a pharmaceutical company's drug prices, their perspective of the industry will most likely have soured over the years.

The costs of drug treatment can vary wildly. From my stints in community pharmacy, I know that some drugs are cheaper than a loaf of bread. On the other hand, there are certain drugs that are simply too expensive for the NHS to fund. NICE[6] has deemed that they just don't

---

[5] NHS – National Health Service, the publicly funded healthcare system in the United Kingdom.

[6] NICE – The National Institute for Health and Clinical Excellence. An independent organisation that supports and advises the National Health Service and social care in the United Kingdom.

tick the "good value for money" box. Particularly in oncology, patients are lined up in order of priority for certain treatments that cost too much to be made freely available on the NHS. In some situations, the clinician has to build a case to justify the patient's eligibility for one of these treatments. They have to prove themselves worthy of being the chosen one – to receive life-saving treatment.

Eculizumab (Soliris) is a humanised mouse monoclonal antibody approved for the treatment of atypical haemolytic uremic syndrome (aHUS) – a rare condition that often quickly leads to kidney and organ failure, which can become life-threatening very quickly[1]. It is the only known effective treatment for aHUS to date, a disease whose triggers and mechanisms are still not completely understood by researchers. Eculizumab's reputation as the world's most expensive drug is hardly surprising when one year's treatment costs approximately $600,000, and aHUS patients require treatment for life[1].

The other members of the monoclonal antibody family are just as guilty of astronomical price points. They might as well have gold in them. Or come packaged in a diamond-encrusted syringe in a gold treasure chest.

Why does this happen? How did the top end of the sliding scale for drug prices disappear so quickly into the clouds?

To understand the pharmaceutical company's reasons for charging these eye-watering figures, let's go through the typical drug development process.

It all starts with identifying a disease area to focus on[2]. For example, GlaxoSmithKline has built a world-leading HIV and respiratory portfolio, whilst Merck has enjoyed considerable success in diabetes treatments over the years. Next, a biological target needs to be identified – when this target is hit by a drug, the resulting effects keep the patient's disease progression and symptoms under control[2].

Now that the target has been identified, a drug can be designed so that it hits the target as selectively and reliably as possible every time it is administered[2]. There are multiple ways to go about this, but high-throughput screening remains a predominant strategy; a fast, automated process that tests whole libraries of potential drug compounds against the chosen target[2].

Think of it as going through your entire bunch of keys one by one when you have no idea which one unlocks your garage door (the biological target). High-throughput screening tests thousands of keys instead, using a robot named Jim who does it exponentially faster than you ever will.

Eventually, several compounds may emerge as potential candidates, also known as leads[2]. These leads now need to be optimised by some very clever medicinal chemists, who manipulate the structure of leads to achieve a specific set of properties. For example, a certain part of the molecule may flip a switch in your body that makes you drowsy when you take the drug. This part of the molecule could be removed, but what if this newly modified molecule triggers another switch that does something else?

I told you they were clever.

Once the lead compound has been nipped and tucked in all the right places, it now needs to go through pre-clinical testing. As the name suggests, initial testing does not happen in humans. Pre-clinical work is typically done in vitro (testing in tissue that has been isolated from an animal or human) and in vivo (testing in live, whole animals). In fact, it is a legal requirement – at least in the UK – that testing takes place in animals before the drug gets anywhere near human trials[12]. The aim is to mimic human conditions as closely as possible, hence the usual choices of animals that closely resemble us on a physiological and anatomical level – rats, dogs and occasionally primates. Tests done here provide valuable information on appropriate dosing and the associated toxicity risks[2]. More importantly, the results from pre-clinical work indicate whether the decision can be made to progress safely to human testing.

Using the information gained from pre-clinical activities, the drug now undergoes pharmaceutical development. This is a great area for pharmacists to roll their sleeves up and get their hands dirty.

Let's say that the decision has been made to formulate drug X as a tablet. The pharmaceutical development team brainstorms the best way to take drug X from a powder on a lab bench to a tablet that can be viably consumed. This includes making decisions on excipient[7] choice, the type of tablet required and the optimal manufacturing process and parameters. When swallowed, this tablet needs to release drug X in a manner that achieves a certain degree of therapeutic benefit.

Most drugs do not come as a pure compound. Sorry to break it to you, but that tablet you take on a daily basis most likely contains more lactose than drug.

The final drug form can now be manufactured on a large scale for use in human clinical trials. When sufficient data is collected from these trials to demonstrate just how promising and revolutionary drug X is,

---

[7] Excipients – the ingredients used in a tablet that do not include the active pharmaceutical ingredient.

the company files for regulatory approval. If everything goes swimmingly, marketing authorisation is granted. Drug X has now been successfully approved by regulatory authorities and is ready to be put on pharmacy shelves.

We got there in the end.

All in all, the process of discovering and developing a drug and getting it to market takes between twelve to fifteen years and can cost up to (and in excess of) $1 billion[2]. To call it an arduous endeavour would be a gross understatement. Each step is time and cost-intensive in its own regard, and to cut down on these expenses equates to compromising patient safety – which should never be an option under any circumstances.

With expenses that accumulate quickly over the years, simple business acumen suggests that the pharmaceutical company needs to recoup their hefty investment somehow. Sure, the drug can be patented to grant the manufacturer a twenty-year period of market exclusivity, during which other companies are excluded from making, using or selling the drug[3]. This gives the original manufacturer a twenty-year monopoly to recoup the costs of developing their drug in exchange for publicly disclosing their invention under the patent[3]. However, this also means that generic drug manufacturers are ready and waiting to swoop in with their cheaper versions of the drug as soon as the patent expires – without having to invest in most of the discovery and development work that the original pharmaceutical company poured into their product.

The most obvious way to recover these costs and maximise the company's return on investment? Charge more for the drug.

Unfortunately, it is often patients who pay the price – so to speak.

The Haggler

Every so often, just as things were starting to fall into a comfortable routine, the Saturday pharmacy staff would be graced with the presence of what I affectionately call "the haggler". You see, the haggler is a special breed of customer you don't meet often. These elusive beings pick their moments. But when they did show up in the pharmacy, they had a habit of getting under my fellow counter assistant's skin to no end – and amusing me to no end.

I had the privilege of serving a haggler one Saturday. Hagglers have a way of looking just like any other customer, but they know exactly how to ensnare you when you least expect it. MI6 could do with their talents. I asked if there was anything I could help with, blissfully unaware of what was to come. This particular haggler wanted a box of paracetamol caplets.

"Sure, that's one pound for the paracetamol caplets," I chirped, making my way over to the till to process the transaction.

He stopped me short and looked at me as if I'd just eaten a baby alive. "One pound?" he said.

"Yes sir, that's one pound."

He looked at me incredulously, mouth agape in shock whilst he desperately fumbled for the right words like a confused goldfish. It didn't feel like the right moment to ask whether he would rather pay by cash or card, so I waited patiently whilst he composed himself.

"This is ridiculous. I could get the same thing for a quarter of the price from the supermarket across the road!"

I could hear the other counter assistant practising his deep breathing exercises.

"I'm sorry sir, but the prices are final. Would you like the paracetamol?"

The haggler seemed to get more and more offended with every word that came out of my mouth. He immediately launched into a lecture on the fundamentals of business strategy and how we were going to bankrupt ourselves if we continued to charge such extortionate prices. How dare we take advantage of decent customers like him, he said. He then threatened to tell anyone who would listen about how awful and immoral this pharmacy's practices were. After a few more TED talks on how to build a profitable business, he declared that he would be buying his paracetamol from the supermarket across the road instead. The door slammed on his way out.

My cheeks hurt from all the smiling. If working in a pharmacy doesn't give you Angelina Jolie cheekbones, I don't know what will.

But the haggler was far from finished. Less than five minutes after he had made his dramatic exit, he was back. His face was an even richer shade of tomato than before. I asked if he still wanted the paracetamol or if there was something else he needed help with.

I was then informed that the supermarket across the street had run out of their generic paracetamol, and nobody in their right mind would be willing to pay close to two pounds for the branded stuff they were selling.

"Just the one box of paracetamol caplets then? That'll be one pound."

I was met yet again with the baby-eater stare. Eyes positively bulging out of his head, he asked, "Well, aren't you going to lower your prices for me?"

Fast-forward through a few more lectures on competitive pricing and customer satisfaction (and more unsuccessful deep breathing exercises from the other counter assistant), the haggler eventually bought the box of paracetamol caplets. He paid the whole pound, fair and square. I could practically see the simmering anger that raged behind his eyes.

Hagglers make me feel alive.

All the Pies

As a Pharmacy student, I never thought the physiological mechanisms of tooth sensitivity would make it into my revision notes. I never thought I'd get the chance to learn about the scientific rationale behind a toothpaste that both whitens teeth and provides protection against that all-too-familiar twinge when I sink my teeth into ice cream.

Yet here we are.

If there is one thing I've learned from the degree I put myself over £35,000 in debt to pursue, it is this – pharmacists have a finger in every pie.

And so they should. Their unique combination of skills puts them in a position that allows them – even encourages them – to explore a diverse buffet of career options.

From a public perspective, community pharmacy may be the apple pie of the pharmacy world – the staple in every household. This is where the pharmacist is most visible after all. However, there is a whole myriad of pies out there that lends itself to a pharmacist's knowledge and skillset. For the modern pharmacist today, the bakery is a very large one indeed.

If being a community pharmacist is the apple pie of pharmacy, working as a hospital pharmacist must be its cousin – the pecan pie. Humble and unassuming, yet belly-warming and bursting with flavour. Pharmacists are a valuable member of the multidisciplinary healthcare team involved in the care of every patient on every hospital ward. I know how much that reeks of "politically correct corporate speak", but that doesn't make it any less true. London's busiest hospitals would fall apart without them.

From the minute you enter the hospital to the last day of your stay, the pharmacist has a say in your care every step of the way. Being the resident drug experts, they decide on an effective drug dosing regimen that won't kill you. Sure, individual NHS trust guidelines and scientific literature aid this decision – but many factors are taken into account; your organ function, past medical history, blood results and patient demographics.

Whilst on placement, I met patients who struggled to swallow normally and thus required nasogastric intubation (a thin plastic tube inserted through the nose down to the stomach). If you happen to be one of these patients, tablets are quite clearly not an option. So, the pharmacist tells the rest of the healthcare team which tablets can be crushed and given down the tube with water, and which ones should be given as a different formulation altogether. If drugs A and B need to be given down that tube together, the pharmacist tells the team whether this can be done safely.

If you happen to need a medicine that isn't regularly used by the hospital, you can bet your bottom dollar that the pharmacist has already read an eye-watering number of research papers on the subject. They are armed with evidence and ready to lobby your case so that you get that damn medicine.

If hospital pharmacy is the pecan pie of the pharmacy careers bakery, the pharmaceutical industry has to be the blackberry pie. Within one pie alone, the options are endless. Top it with toasted meringue, ice cream, whipped cream or enjoy it with no topping at all. The filling is a whole other ball game – blackberry and apple, add raspberry or strawberries, or just blackberries and blackberries only.

In other words, there are numerous roles within the pharmaceutical industry that welcome pharmacists with open arms. A pharmacist can work in drug safety and pharmacovigilance, which revolves around monitoring, assessing and understanding the adverse effects of a medicine[4]. This is very much a priority for any pharmaceutical company – clinical trials only demonstrate the effects of the drug in a relatively small patient population. The longer a drug has been on the market, the higher the volume of data that can be gathered on the severity and frequency of adverse events experienced by patients on a global scale.

By analysing drug safety data, potential risk factors and patient populations who are vulnerable to these adverse effects can be identified. This in turn informs required regulatory actions and enables more relevant, engaging communication of safety information to physicians and patients. It therefore goes without saying that pharmacovigilance work is a crucial part of post-marketing surveillance. Pharmacists have an advantage in this department thanks to their specialist knowledge of drug effects and clinical expertise.

Quality assurance is another area that lends itself to a pharmacist's meticulous, detail-oriented nature. Manufacturing drug products to a consistently high standard is the name of the game; any deviations from this standard could result in product defects and patients ultimately suffer the consequences. The quality stream in the pharmaceutical industry ensures that the manufacturing processes are validated and testing is conducted and documented to regulatory standards – so that the product reaches the patient exactly as promised.

Pharmaceutical science is a significant element of a pharmacist's training, which opens up Research and Development (R&D) doors should they wish to go down that route. A pharmacist's training equips them with the knowledge required to get involved in many aspects of drug discovery and formulation. Always wondered why some medicines only exist as tablets whereas others come as creams, inhalers and various other formulations? This is just one of the many decisions made by R&D that require careful consideration of all sorts of variables.

Take the patient experience, for instance. Ever been pleasantly surprised by a tablet that tastes nice? This is most likely the result of a decision that was made specifically with you – the consumer – in mind. If people don't like the taste of their medicines, they associate the medicine with a negative experience and may be less likely to adhere to their doctor's instructions. It logically follows that if a tasty coating is added, these same people are more likely to associate their medicine with a positive experience and take their medicines more diligently. Everyone wins.

Occasionally, you'll meet a particularly nosy breed of pharmacist who wants to keep a finger in the pharmaceutical pie, the academic pie and the clinical pie all at the same time. These characters are perfect for the medical science liaison (MSL) role. MSLs serve as a bridge between clinicians, researchers at academic institutions and pharmaceutical companies. They provide scientific expertise in the context of a drug's clinical use, and they tend to be excellent communicators who have the ability to explain anything to anyone. True to their nosy trait, MSLs are often very interested in emerging clinical trends, and will most likely be in the know of the latest research and new developments within their specialty.

All pie analogies aside, I hope I managed to offer you a peek into the diversity of careers available to a Pharmacy graduate. As someone very wise once told me, "Studying Pharmacy prepares you for so much more than being a pharmacist."

Please excuse me whilst I go satisfy my self-induced hankering for pie.

Hair Dye and Lady Business

Being the only female member of the Saturday pharmacy staff came with its perks. Many of the regular customers tended to visit the pharmacy to browse the cosmetic counters, and I had somehow been dubbed the resident beauty consultant. All questions remotely hair and beauty-related were immediately flung in my direction like a hot coal.

Looking back, I should have asked for a pay rise. Choosing between "ivory" and "porcelain" foundation to match Karen's skin tone was definitely not discussed in the interview. Maybe it had just been very expertly hidden in the fine print of my contract.

The afternoon lull had begun on yet another Saturday, when a lady walked in asking for hair dye. I pointed her in the direction of the hair dye shelves and left her to browse in peace, whilst I got on with pricing the remainder of the new stock that had arrived that morning. Moments later, she was back at the counter.

"What do you think, darling? Honey blonde or ice blonde?"

Either would flatter her, but ice blonde may be a little more difficult to maintain – I responded without skipping a beat. A purple shampoo or a toner of some kind might be necessary to keep those nasty orange tones at bay and maintain the desired ashy hue. The ice blonde would really bring out the cool blue shade of her eyes too.

Disclaimer - I've dabbled in hair colouring a few times myself, but I'm no John Frieda. Please ask your stylist for professional advice.

By now, the other two male pharmacy staff had eavesdropped on enough of the conversation to be satisfied that this customer was being dealt with. They promptly retreated behind the counter to begin their own discussion of last night's Prime Minister's Questions over a cup of tea. At this point, the woman put both boxes of hair dye down and turned to me.

"Can I ask you... a lady question?" she ventured hesitantly, her voice lowered to a whisper.

She confessed that she needed some advice on some symptoms she had been experiencing "down there". She had never experienced anything like it before, and it had been troubling her for a while. With some gentle encouragement on my part, she described what sounded like classic symptoms of thrush and asked if there was anything she could buy over the counter to get rid of it. As it was her first time experiencing these symptoms, I apologised that I couldn't sell her anything until she had visited her GP to get a confirmed diagnosis. I assured her that this was perfectly normal and very common.

She exhaled a sigh of relief that she must have been holding in since she walked through the door, and thanked me over and over. She was so grateful that there was someone in the pharmacy she could talk to about these things without – in her words, "dying of embarrassment". Needless to say, I was overflowing with the warm fuzzies as I thanked her for allowing me to help.

Sometimes, taking care of a patient is about the little things – that are, in many ways, the biggest things. There is no golden formula that works every time. Getting a patient to tell you what you need to know is nothing like the box-ticking exercise they use in clinical practice classes to teach us patient consultation skills. Wearing a white coat or a badge with "Pharmacist" on it does not automatically entitle you to the information you require from patients. Information that patients often want to tell you, but may not always be able to do so without a little nudge.

If I remember correctly, I believe she went with ice blonde.

Essential Oils or Essentially Quackery?

I am of the opinion that if it works, it works. The end. We all live happily ever after.

The subject of herbal medicine – more specifically, its plausibility as a medicine – boasts an undefeated talent for sparking impassioned debates where temperatures often rise quickly. Personally, I am most familiar with conventional medicine based on evidence-based practice. I take comfort in knowing that the medicines I will be working with as a pharmacist are heavily regulated, and they will all have run the gauntlet of rigorous multiphase clinical trials. On the other hand, I grew up with herbal medicine. Herbal soups and traditional Chinese remedies were a normal part of daily life. Some of my earliest memories include being fed a concoction of a highly aromatic brown powder dissolved in water, whose "cooling" properties – I was told – would get rid of my sore throat.

But hey – it if works, it works.

Herbal medicine is defined as plant-based medicine used to treat disease or maintain good health, typically made from differing combinations of plant parts[5].

"Wait a minute, doesn't digoxin come from foxglove too?"

Correct. Digoxin is a drug commonly used in the management of arrhythmias (abnormal heart rhythms) and it is indeed extracted from foxglove leaves. However, the main difference lies in the fact that it is isolated and purified as a single chemical compound to form a highly pure product[6]. Herbal medicine, on the other hand, tends to use whole plants or whole plant parts in the form of extracts that have not been purified[5,8]. These extracts can be obtained from either fresh or dried plant matter, depending on the herb in question[5].

Why do people use herbal medicine? All sorts of reasons. In countries where healthcare is privatised, herbal medicine may be a more affordable option compared to conventional medicine. Patients may have suffered such a negative experience with conventional medicine in the past that they would rather avoid it altogether. In some cases, a patient receives a diagnosis where conventional medicine is no longer effective. They may seek out alternative medicine as a last resort, or as a means of pain relief if nothing else. Other reasons can include cultural beliefs and easier access to herbal medicines.

Popping into Holland and Barrett's on your local high street takes significantly less time than waiting for a doctor's appointment. It is a fact that just isn't worth disputing.

Regardless of our opinion of the patient's decisions regarding their healthcare, we are taught to respect the patient's autonomy. Whether we agree with their choice or not is irrelevant. Offering objective advice is all we can do, and all we should do.

That being said, there are several particularly intriguing pieces of objective advice regarding herbal medicine that I have learned over the years. I'd like to take this opportunity to share them with you.

Let's start with the legal stuff, the epitome of "objective advice". In the UK, the herbal medicines available in pharmacies are most likely to have been granted either one of two things – a product license or a Traditional Herbal Registration (THR) number under the Traditional Herbal Medicine Registration Scheme (THMRS)[7]. A herbal product is granted a product license only if there is sufficient evidence to demonstrate its efficacy as a medicine – therefore making it worthy of full marketing authorisation status, just like conventional medicines.

What about the herbal medicines with THR numbers? Have they demonstrated efficacy?

The short answer is no. A herbal medicine does not need to prove clinical efficacy to be granted a Traditional Herbal Registration[7,8]. Sure, their quality and safety will have been assessed by the MHRA (Medicines and Healthcare products Regulatory Agency) - the UK's regulatory highness that regulates medicines, medical devices and blood components for transfusion. They ensure that these products contain the listed ingredient, the correct dose of said listed ingredient and have not been compromised in quality by the addition of heavy metals, pharmaceutical materials or nasty substances we really shouldn't ingest[7]. However, no proof of efficacy is required in the form of clinical trial results or preclinical results[8]. None. Nada.

In short, this means that these products can be successfully registered under the THMRS without having undergone testing in humans. This is perhaps the biggest difference between a herbal medicine registered under the THMRS and a conventional medicine with a product licence.

Why the fuss about efficacy? Why is efficacy such an important buzzword in medicine? Well, efficacy is a measure of the therapeutic response achieved by a drug in lab studies or clinical trials, which translates into the degree of success the drug achieves in managing a patient's disease[11]. In essence – how well the drug works.

This is not to say that efficacy is completely unaccounted for in herbal medicines registered under the THMRS. Efficacy and permitted indications (uses) for these products are determined based on their "traditional use" instead of data from research studies – where "traditional use" is defined by the product having been used for medicinal purposes for at least thirty years, including at least fifteen years within the European community[8].

If it works, it works.

Herbal medicine is just one branch of the broader canopy of complementary and alternative medicine (CAM). "Complementary" indicates treatments that are used alongside standard medical treatments – for example, acupuncture to relieve side effects of cancer treatment. "Alternative" refers to treatments that are used in the place of standard medical treatments altogether. What about the people who practice CAM? Who are they?

The General Regulatory Council for Complementary Therapies states that regulation and registration of complementary therapists in the

UK is via voluntary self-regulation[9]. They go on to state explicitly that "there are no laws in place to protect the public from unqualified or incompetent therapists"[9].

If it works, it works.

Herbal medicines are often associated with keywords like "gentle" and "natural", which tend to be very good at evoking imagery of a dense green forest where foliage stretches as far as the eye can see – not dissimilar to the kind featured in those disarmingly seductive Herbal Essences shampoo commercials. However, there is a reason healthcare professionals are taught to ask if you take any herbal medicines. Herbal remedies can interact with prescription medicines – interfering with their pharmacological action and potentially causing all sorts of undesirable effects. St. John's Wort is a known repeat offender in the drug interactions arena. It clashes with all sorts of drugs under the sun - from oral contraceptives and antidepressants to warfarin and HIV antiretrovirals[10]. Believe it or not, the innocent-looking garlic and ginkgo biloba have their own criminal records too[10].

I'll keep it short. If you take any herbal medicines or plan to start, let your doctor or pharmacist know. They'll want to hear about it, I promise.

Personally, until stricter regulations are enforced on the supply of herbal products and a more comprehensive evidence base is required by law to demonstrate their efficacy, I think I'll keep my relationship with herbs strictly on a kitchen cupboard level for now. They seem quite happy there.

Peach and basil desserts, anyone?

Professional Pedantry

The unfortunate souls who have gotten to know me well over the years will tell you that I am first and foremost a pedant. The worst thing about this is perhaps the fact that I take pride in identifying as one. So much so, that I took a year out of Pharmacy school to gain experience in being pedantic for a living.

On my CV, this is written as "Validation experience in the pharmaceutical industry", but don't be fooled.

Between my penultimate and final years at university, I embarked on a year of work experience in the world of pharmaceutical supply and manufacturing. This was the first time I had worked full time and lived independently, and the learning curve was – at times – an uncomfortably steep one. I learned how to budget to the penny with the help of my embarrassingly basic Excel spreadsheet. I learned that meal prepping was the best way to curb my nightly garlic bread cravings. I realised that I was extremely competitive in post-work exercise classes, where all the Karens and Tracies had triceps that made mine look like overcooked noodles.

Aside from a crash course on how to navigate adult life, I learned about the role of the Quality stream in a pharmaceutical company. I immersed myself in all things QbD (Quality by Design) and GMP (Good Manufacturing Practice), along with other keywords I'd only ever heard mentioned fleetingly in university lectures. I was thrilled to meet other pharmacists in this line of work, who helped me recognise the value of having a clinical perspective in pharmaceutical manufacturing.

I spent those twelve months in Quality Assurance, specifically in the Validation department. Validation is the practice of demonstrating that a piece of equipment is capable of reproducing the expected results to the same standard every time. In proper speak, this piece of equipment needs to "consistently demonstrate compliance with regulatory standards". This is achieved by designing and executing a testing protocol according to GMP standards[8], and documenting evidence throughout the testing process. In turn, the evidence is used to build a complete audit trail to show that the piece of equipment can indeed produce the desired results every time.

---

[8] GMP standards – According to the FDA, GMP standards define the minimum requirements for the methods, facilities and controls used in the manufacturing, processing and packing of a drug product.

As a colleague once said, "If it ain't written down, it didn't happen."

Why is validation important in drug manufacture? Well, to put it simply – without validation, there is no way to tell whether every batch of a drug that reaches patients is of the same, high quality. For example, one inhaler dose may contain less active pharmaceutical ingredient than another due to a manufacturing inconsistency or defect. Without quality assurance to spot this, there is a risk that the patient may be under-dosing and thus not getting adequate disease management.

The FDA[9] and other regulatory agencies need to know that the final drug product meets its specification. More importantly, they need to know that this is the case only because a system has been developed and tested to reliably produce batches that will all successfully meet specifications.

Unlike home baking, validation ensures that every batch of cupcakes is baked to perfection every time – where "perfection" is defined by a set of very specific criteria. There is no tolerance for lumpy batter, overfilling or under-baking in the world of pharmaceutical drug manufacture.

---

[9] FDA – US Food and Drug Administration regulates food, drugs, cosmetics and other medical products to protect public health and safety.

Validation itself is a broad concept that can be applied to much more than pieces of equipment. Manufacturing processes need to be validated to confirm that the product meets its specification when manufactured within defined critical process parameters. Cleaning processes following the manufacture of specific products need to be validated to ensure that the next product manufactured is not contaminated by residue from the previous product. I had the opportunity to dabble in these areas as the validation representative within project teams. Project meetings frequently included engineers, technologists and another quality representative.

Working in validation taught me several things about myself. Being the person in charge of quality oversight, I found myself playing the nit-picker who spotted the little things; deviations, documentation errors and whatnot. Though these little things would not have remained so little if swept under the carpet, and sweeping anything under the carpet was a big no-no in itself. I was the person who had to ask the engineers and technicians to re-execute testing, and tell production teams that a certain piece of equipment was going to be out of use for yet another week because of said re-testing.

Let's put it this way – engineering didn't like me much.

I discovered that I loved working in validation. Being someone who, quite frankly, had no idea what validation was when I accepted the job, I found out that it was a great fit for me and my detail-oriented nature. The projects I worked on may not have required a great deal of clinical knowledge, but being a pharmacist in training helped me see the bigger picture. My understanding of basic pharmaceutical manufacturing helped me understand the necessity for the validation rationale behind certain manufacturing processes or cleaning methods. My knowledge of the patient perspective helped me make challenging decisions and always put patient safety first.

A few months after my year in industry ended, I was back at university to complete my final year of the MPharm degree. For me, this kicked off with spending three months working on my research project in industry. Industry-academia partnerships specific to my university enabled truly unique research experiences for a selected few students, and I was lucky enough to be one of them.

Since my project involved extensive testing of inhalers, I found myself spending a great deal of time in the company labs. Getting to work at half past seven in the morning and being the last to leave in the evenings became my new routine. But as far as I was concerned, I had nothing to complain about – I had the opportunity to conduct research in the field of respiratory drug delivery, something I had always been passionate about. I enjoyed commandeering my own project, and I had good support from my supervisors. Every workday ended with a slobbery welcome from my landlady's loving dogs. I was happy.

Ironically, I also found myself receiving the other end of the Quality stick. As this particular company specialised in quality assurance expertise, all pharmaceutical testing and analysis work was done to GMP standards. In a nutshell, things had to be done a very particular way in their labs.

All of a sudden, I had gone from being the nagger to the nagged. The lab quality staff paid me a visit every five minutes – at least that's what it felt like when I was working to deadlines tighter than my skinniest jeans – where I was inundated with requests to update paperwork, asked where procedure X had been documented, and so forth. All very similar questions I myself had posed to the engineers and technicians in my previous role. They were just as unrelenting as they were eagle-eyed.

My former colleague's words taunted me, "If it ain't written down, it didn't happen."

Here's the thing. Having experienced both sides of the Quality coin in the pharmaceutical industry, I can still confidently say that I would love a career in pharmaceutical Quality Assurance someday. Maybe that's what I'll do when I grow up – that is, before I decide I've had enough and can retire comfortably in a lake house with my army of dogs.

Until then, it might just be a life of professional pedantry for me. And I'm not mad about it.

How to Annoy Your Pharmacist

Some pharmacists can be prickly, cynical creatures. However - like most prickly, cynical creatures – a soft heart is usually guarded very closely beneath the tough exterior. They tend to put their patients' best interests first and will do almost anything and fight almost anyone to ensure that their patients receive the treatment they need.

Nevertheless, there are certain customers who seem to take pleasure in poking at this prickly hide. Some don't even realise they do it. They tend to be remarkably persistent, too. If they're not careful, it's only a matter of time until they drive their frazzled pharmacist to do the unthinkable.

Make these customers wait an extra five minutes for their prescription. I know, the sheer audacity.

I can hear your shocked gasps from here. What could these customers possibly be doing that ruffles the poor pharmacist's feathers so effectively? Courtesy of yours truly, here are just a few tried and tested techniques you can put to the test yourself the next time you pick up a prescription. I have witnessed these in action and I am intimately familiar with their feather-ruffling powers. Use at your own peril.

You also didn't hear them from me.

Customers asking to see the pharmacist regarding a medical query are not uncommon. This forms an integral part of a pharmacist's training, and they will usually be quite happy to help you dispel (or confirm) any fears you had when you walked in. Ask your question and allow your pharmacist to offer their explanation, giving them an occasional nod to indicate that you are listening. However, every so often, interrupt them loudly whilst they are still speaking. It helps to throw in medical jargon that has nothing to do with the discussion at hand – even better if you have absolutely no idea what it means yourself.

If this doesn't satisfy your prickly skin-prodding urges, play the herbal card. When picking up your prescription, make a point to disparage modern evidence-based medicine as aggressively as you can. Spice it up for the audience by singing the praises of garlic supplements and essential oils. If you're committed to selling it, maybe start an impromptu monologue on why "natural is best". Make sure to passionately address the fact that pharmaceutical companies deserve all the slander they get for forcing "all the nasty chemicals" down our throats and milking our bank accounts dry.

I received this very same monologue not in a pharmacy, but over a Tinder chat. We never made it beyond Tinder.

Pharmacists won't tell you this, but they enjoy a good prank every now and then. Feel free to indulge them – all work and no play makes Jack a very dull pharmacist after all. Storm into the pharmacy on a particularly busy day, allowing the door to swing wide on its hinges behind you. In your whiniest, most grating voice, demand to collect your repeat prescription – wait for it – when you haven't ordered one in the first place.

If the counter assistant is anywhere near as conflict averse as I am, you may be met with a gentle stream of apologies as they desperately search the shelves whilst cursing under their breath. If they are feeling particularly feisty that day, they may suggest that you double-check whether you have submitted a request for a repeat prescription in the first place. Of course, no matter what they tell you, refute it indignantly – and don't forget to look offended. The pharmacist may never say it, but this little display will make their day and they secretly enjoy a little drama from time to time.

If you're looking for something truly extraordinary for a special occasion, look no further. Your pharmacist deserves to be spoiled, and I have the perfect solution. When your prescription is ready to be collected, ask your pharmacist why it takes them so long to stick "a bloody label" on a box.

If your pharmacist's eyes haven't turned into throbbing cartoon hearts by now, I'm afraid I'm out of pointers.

I lied, I have one left. Use it wisely.

Occasionally, the pharmacist may offer a brief explanation of what your drug does and how it helps your condition when you collect a prescription. If this is a new drug for you, they may invite you to have a tête-à-tête in the private consultation room as part of the New Medicines Service. This conversation is an opportunity for them to cover important points concerning the drug that you should be aware of before starting therapy. When they have finished telling you about your new medication, they will – hopefully – open the floor for any questions you may have at this point.

Say that you'd rather take said questions to your doctor. Thank them for their time. Turn on your heel and walk out immediately for maximum effect.

You can thank me later.

The Ones Who Don't Help Themselves

From refusals to take a medicine due to an unappealing colour to overenthusiastic offers to show me their hernia, patients can be mystifying creatures. When I was told that no two days in healthcare would ever be the same, it was no marketing gimmick for school careers fairs. They were being as literal as it gets.

It's almost as if patients plan these things. "If we work together and time it right, the pharmacy staff *will* lose their minds."

Perhaps I should preface this by clarifying that when all is said and done, a good healthcare professional always wants the best for their patients. No matter how bumpy the ride gets along the way, all they want is a happy and healthy patient at the end of it.

Medication non-adherence is a very real issue that costs the NHS a significant amount in wasted medication every year. Medication gets dispensed, the patient doesn't take it, it gets stockpiled until it eventually goes out of date and ends up back in the dispensary – in the medicines waste bin. When a prescription is handed over to the patient, an assumption is made that they will take the medication as instructed by their doctor or pharmacist. At least most of the time; patients are only human and we are well aware that it is unrealistic to expect perfect compliance from every patient. It is perfectly normal to forget a pill every so often, and we are trained to anticipate this. There is a reason for including the "What to do if you miss a dose" section in patient information leaflets after all.

But sometimes, a few too many pills are forgotten. Or the medication doesn't make it out of the packaging at all.

Occasionally, there will be patients who don't take their medicines at home despite having been provided with all the right supplies and information. This could be intentional non-adherence, where the patient actively chooses not to take their medicines due to personal beliefs or preferences. In short, reasons that are not for us to judge.

In some situations, it may be a case of unintentional non-adherence, where the patient is unable to take their medicines as directed. A patient may have arthritis so severe that they cannot pop tablets out of the foil packaging, or someone may have coordination difficulties that prevent them from using an inhaler correctly. Nevertheless, the result is the same – the medicine doesn't get taken as directed.

On the other hand, some will happily fool their doctor and pharmacist into believing that they have been taking their medicines diligently since day one. Sometimes, I get to witness an Oscar-worthy performance where patients still collect repeat prescriptions on time every month – despite not taking the medicines as they should at home. This is something my hamster brain struggles to comprehend.

Your pharmacist doesn't want a façade of the perfect patient. They are much more interested in the reason you don't take your medicines in the first place.

Drugs don't work if you don't take them. Your pharmacist's priority is your health and wellbeing, and they would much rather know the truth so that they can work with you to find a solution. Unpleasant side effects can often be managed. There may be other options if you find tablets difficult to swallow. If you disagree with your diagnosis altogether and think there is something else going on, your pharmacist wants to know. If you think your pharmacist isn't qualified to help you with a particular issue, they want to know too – so that they can find someone who is. A problem that is not addressed cannot be solved.

Smoking cessation services are a common offering in most community pharmacies, and can be a great resource to give someone the push they need to quit smoking for good. I distinctly remember a certain feisty respiratory consultant pharmacist who delivered one of my favourite lectures at university. Her passion (must have been the Scottish accent) was so contagious that she made a three-hour lecture feel like a private counselling session with Barack Obama himself.

Face the consequences of your patient's smoking habit with them, she said. They'll respect you more for having the balls to do it. I walked out of that lecture feeling like Superman.

She also told us that smoking increases your risk of developing COPD twenty-fold. COPD is a chronic respiratory condition where patients suffer from breathlessness and a persistent cough. Smoking tends to significantly accelerate disease progression as well as the decline of a patient's lung function. In its later stages, it can be severely debilitating.

However, COPD is only a fraction of the smoking picture. There are people much better qualified than I am who can tell you that smoking also predisposes you to things like lung cancer, recurring respiratory tract infections and a whole host of other equally delightful maladies.

People smoke for all sorts of reasons – hell, some healthcare professionals smoke themselves. However, it baffles me that despite the array of options offered by the NHS to help them kick the habit, there are patients who continue to smoke undeterred – in full knowledge of the consequences.

Perhaps I hold this stance on these patients because I am only familiar with one side of the coin. The shiny, polished side only familiar to someone who has never had to take prescription medicines on a lifelong basis for a chronic condition. Someone who has been told all her life that "smoking is bad", someone whose lips have never touched a cigarette. Someone who has never had to grapple with drug addiction whilst being surrounded by disapproving grimaces when society catches a whiff of cigarette smoke on their clothes.

It is easier to categorise certain patients as the black sheep who don't help themselves. It is much easier to put them in a box than to ask why these patients don't behave in a way we expect. Maybe the real question we should be asking is what healthcare professionals can do better to help these patients help themselves.

Warm Healthcare Fuzzies

"Multidisciplinary team" is a hot buzzword that gets thrown around in healthcare like bird seed to the rabid pigeons in London's St. James' Park. As a student, I was made aware on many occasions that I should be working collaboratively with professionals from other healthcare disciplines to ensure that the patient receives the highest possible standard of care.

So many buzzwords.

Remember those interprofessional education sessions? They were designed for this exact purpose; to teach us to work together to achieve the common goal of improving the patient's health and wellbeing. Only with the added excitement of playing The Sims with patient scenarios.

Despite everyone in the room being a healthcare student of some kind, it usually dawned on everyone in the first five minutes or so just how little we knew about each other's courses – and each other. I learned that nursing students spend a great deal of time on placement, and twelve-hour shifts at the hospital as a student are not uncommon. I found out that the dental students have a special simulation room filled with dental mannequin heads that they get to practice on. Those things would serve disarmingly well as horror film props.

"Play with dental heads" is now officially on my bucket list.

Several medics and I got talking about OSCEs (objective structured clinical examinations), and they were surprised to learn that Pharmacy students had to run the gauntlet of OSCEs too, just like themselves. The OSCE is the highly anticipated (or dreaded) clinical exam at the end of every academic year, designed to assess practical skills in a simulated clinical setting. It tends to be split into a series of short stations that test a specific set of skills required for each healthcare discipline. For pharmacists, this can range from handling clinical problems to resolving law-related prescription issues.

My personal favourite has to be the station that tests patient consultation skills with the help of an actor, who plays a patient with a medical query that you need to solve whilst maintaining a calm, professional manner.

Confession - I've always wanted to play a stubborn, difficult patient whose mission is to make the healthcare professional's life hell, though

I think I might enjoy it a bit too much. As it turns out, the medics actually have to deal with this in their OSCEs. One of their stations involves dealing with a "challenging" patient, and they are scored based on how they handle the situation.

I don't think I would make it through two minutes of that patient consultation without my head exploding volcano style – you know, like they do in cartoons.

I also learned that when on placement, nursing students are expected to conduct routine blood tests on patients. They are so highly skilled that their supervisors entrust them with these tasks without batting an eye. If I had to take someone's blood, I think I would spend a good few minutes alone trying to get the gloves over my shaking, hopelessly sweaty hands whilst withering under the patient's perplexed stare.

The sweatier your hands are, the more difficult it is to get those gloves on. The more I struggle with the gloves, the more my hands sweat. It's the most vicious of vicious cycles.

I haven't even reached the part where the patient becomes my personal pincushion.

Then, the two nursing students in my group said something I did not expect to hear. They told me how much respect they had for the pharmacists on their hospital placements. They told me all about how knowledgeable these pharmacists were and how reliable they were when other healthcare professionals had a drug-related query. I was asked about the nature of my clinical training and how pharmacists could possibly retain so much information about every drug. Whilst they continued to sing the praises of the pharmacists they had met, I sat there speechless with delight. I couldn't believe it. I simply had no words.

Those nursing students made my day. For the first time, I was truly proud to call myself a pharmacist-in-training.

Friends in Shady Places

I google my symptoms.

I know, I know. I tell people not to do it, but I can't resist doing it myself. In fact, I've been known to frequent Wikipedia more than I'd like to admit. I like to think of it as the ever warm and welcoming opium den of revision resources. It seduces me with its dimly lit alcoves that harbour the juicy secrets to nailing my university coursework. It whispers sweet nothings in my ear and tempts me with promises of enlightenment. And yes, it leaves me satisfied.

I am also guilty of visiting its cousin every so often – WebMD. Headache that seems a little too persistent? WebMD. Sore throat that has been going on for a while and doesn't seem to be getting any better? WebMD. Friend asking about a urinary tract infection? WebMD.

Sometimes, resources that have a more unsavoury reputation in the eyes of the academic community provide a simple and accurate explanation – exactly what I need. Pharmacy school would be more aptly named "Daily Information Overload" on the glossy university brochures aimed at hopeful sixteen-year-olds. Being bombarded with complex concepts in overwhelming detail was something that I had to learn to deal with very early on. Learning and retaining absolutely everything in four years' worth of lectures was simply impossible.

And it is. Pharmacists don't know it all.

I was once on placement in a tertiary care centre, where I had a wonderful supervising pharmacist who took time out of her schedule to discuss patient cases with me. We had come across a medical term on a patient's chart whose definition had momentarily slipped our minds. She said three words that made me feel like an acne-ridden teenager who had just been handed a box of condoms.

"Just google it."

I wasted no time. A few seconds later, we had found our answer and had moved on to discussing the pharmacokinetics of the next drug on the chart. However, that moment stuck with me. Every so often, as it turns out, professionals google things too. That little search bar isn't some shady corner reserved for the black sheep of the student population – the ones who don't run straight to the "proper" textbooks and journals for the answers. The ones who just need to take a step back to simplify everything. The ones who want to fully understand basic concepts before they think about approaching the high and mighty textbooks and journals.

I am one of these black sheep. Sometimes, my hamster brain just needs some help from the more unconventional resources. Khan Academy, here I come.

Unpopular Opinions

Treat your patient as a complete human being, they say. The patient in front of you is a person, not a condition. "Patient-centred healthcare" is quite literally the first core concept in "Medicines, Ethics and Practice" – the bible on all things pharmacy ethics and legislation, courtesy of the Royal Pharmaceutical Society.

I mean, they're not wrong. Besides actual medical knowledge, ethics is probably the star quarterback of healthcare. It has a prominent role in every patient's care, whether they need paracetamol for a tension headache or palliative care in end-stage renal disease. It's here to stay.

As part of our training, simulated patient scenarios are common teaching tools that help prepare us for the real world of clinical practice. The aim of the game is to get us to apply the clinical knowledge gained over the course of the degree to making a decision concerning a patient's healthcare. Giving us a taste of flying before pushing us out of the nest, if you will. The ethics patient scenarios often featured an ethical dilemma that required us to decide on the best course of action

82

for the patient in question. A particularly memorable one I encountered went a little something like this.

You are the responsible pharmacist in XYZ Pharmacy. It is a Friday evening and a man gives you a prescription for his mother for oxycodone tablets. She has cancer, and you know the man well as he regularly collects his mother's medicines from your pharmacy. This time, he seems distressed as his mother has taken a turn for the worse since starting chemotherapy. You check the prescription to find that the prescriber's signature is missing. After explaining this to the man, he volunteers to go back to the GP[10] surgery to get it signed as his mother has run out of oxycodone at home. Although you know the surgery is about five miles away, he insists that he can drive there to get the prescription signed by the doctor and make it back in time to get the medicines dispensed. Twenty minutes later, your dispenser takes in the same prescription. It is now signed, but the signature is not one you recognise. You try ringing the GP surgery to query this, but you get the surgery's closed message. What do you do?

Before we delve into the issues in this case, there are a few things I should mention. Firstly, it is illegal for a pharmacist to dispense a prescription missing the prescriber's signature. The pharmacist cannot sign a prescription on the prescriber's behalf. There is no real

---

[10] GP – General Practitioner

alternative here except to chase down the prescriber and politely ask through gritted teeth if they could pretty please sign the damn thing.

Secondly, there are certain medicines that can be dispensed without a prescription in an emergency – a possible way out of this scenario. Provided that the circumstances and the patient fulfil certain criteria, this is a decision that typically falls to the professional judgment of the pharmacist. However, the oxycodone tablets this man wants are classified as a Schedule 2 Controlled Drug (CD)[11]. Schedule 2 CDs are most definitely not on the "okay" list for emergency prescriptions. Therefore, this immediately rules out the option of giving him the tablets as an emergency prescription.

The main issue here is the possibility of a fraudulent prescription. Doing a ten-mile return trip in twenty minutes is perfectly possible. Mathematically speaking, he would have had to be driving at a speed of 30 mph at the very least – not to mention allowing time to park the car, get the prescription signed, and make it back to the pharmacy in Friday rush hour traffic. Unlikely, but not impossible.

---

[11] The misuse of Drugs Regulations 2001 divided drugs into five Schedules, each specifying the requirements for importing, exporting, possession, prescribing and record keeping of drugs according to each Schedule.

However, the signature was also one the pharmacist did not recognise – cue alarm bells. Getting the surgery's closed message on the phone only heightens suspicion.

Dispensing medication from a fraudulent prescription is illegal and there was no way of checking the validity of the signature until the following Monday. After considerable debate, there were only two real options. The pharmacist could refuse to dispense the oxycodone, leaving the man's mother with no pain relief all weekend. Alternatively, the pharmacist could take a gamble and dispense the oxycodone regardless. In the slim chance that the signature turned out to be valid, everybody wins. If the signature turned out to be false, the pharmacist would have no choice but to kiss their career goodbye and get comfortable in prison for a long, long time.

Following the discussion with the lecturer and the rest of the year group, the general consensus emerged - the pharmacist should refuse to dispense the oxycodone, and withhold the potentially fraudulent prescription for safekeeping. They should record details of the incident and direct the man to NHS 111[12] before calling the GP surgery again the following Monday to query the signature.

---

[12] NHS 111 is a 24-hour service provided by the NHS over the phone or online for patients with an urgent medical query. Depending on the situation, the patient can be advised on what local services are available or connected directly to a nurse, emergency dentist, GP or pharmacist for advice.

I'm not sure what your thoughts are, but this didn't sit right with me. Sure, I'm all for record keeping and flagging a fake signature, but there is a bigger problem here.

By refusing to dispense the oxycodone, the pharmacist is actively choosing to leave the man's mother in pain over the weekend.

It is easy to promote patient-centred care as a high-level guiding principle. However, when it comes to everyday practice, the correct decision is often unclear. In fact, there may be no correct decision. For the sake of protecting themselves, the pharmacist in this scenario had to forego their first and foremost duty for the sake of legality; looking after the patient's wellbeing. We may not have known the patient's stage of disease or the degree of pain she was in – she may have been able to cope without oxycodone for two days. But this should have had zero bearing on whether the healthcare professional decides to prioritise her welfare or not.

You could argue that the pharmacist did suggest that the patient call NHS 111. They didn't exactly drop all responsibility like a hot coal and send the patient away with nothing.

But they were in a position to help.

Dialling 111 comes with the same degree of uncertainty, and the man may have been similarly unsuccessful there. The pharmacist had been presented with a very real, tangible opportunity to help the patient. Sure, it came with many strings attached - I would not blame any pharmacist for refusing to dispense the oxycodone in this scenario. But the instinct to play hot potato with responsibility when the situation gets sticky doesn't help matters. Sure, the legislation isn't written to benefit every scenario and in this case, the law only encourages the hot potato game. But since when did protecting ourselves at all costs take precedence – and become our first instinct – over prioritising a patient's welfare?

In short, today's unpopular opinion – more action, less arse coverage.

The Bare Necessities

As anyone who works in the retail industry will tell you, a customer-facing role seems to be a hotbed for weird and wonderful characters. I say this with love - Mr. B was definitely one of the regular visitors who were more weird than they were wonderful.

The first time we met, I was fairly wet behind the ears and was still getting to know my way around my job at the pharmacy. When it came to the regular patients, I was just as blissfully clueless as you are. All the female pharmacy staff had given me good-natured warnings about him, but I clearly had no idea what was really in store for me.

It was ten minutes from closing time on a Saturday evening. I had just given the counters a wipe down, but there seemed to be a perpetual sticky layer of – I won't finish that sentence. Whilst I scrubbed away in an attempt to kill time, the bell on the door tinkled. I looked up to see Mr. B hobbling in on his trusty walking stick. Wearing my best customer service smile, I asked how I could assist him today.

88

He wanted to collect his prescription, he said. After confirming his details and asking the usual questions, I handed it over. He immediately proceeded to open the paper bag, searching through the medicines for a good few seconds with his eyebrows furrowed in deep concentration. Concerned that there might have been a dispensing error, I asked if he was missing anything.

"There it is," he said as he produced the box of Viagra with a triumphant flourish. "Oh, I've needed this. You know what I mean, don't you darling?" he said with a sly smirk, waggling his eyebrows at me.

I do know what you mean, Mr. B – though I wish I didn't. So that's what all the well-meaning warnings were about. The mobility of those eyebrows was astonishing. Truly. Whilst I stood there, still frozen to the spot trying to process what I had just witnessed, he took his sweet time repacking the bag before he left – but not before giving me an exaggerated wink on his way out.

As far as eyebrows go, I don't think I've ever encountered a more memorable pair. I hope you're still enjoying the finer things in life, pal.

Flying the Pharmacy Flag

A very clever friend of mine once said, "Pharmacists just need a massive ego boost, you know?"

He was referring to the unspoken hierarchy that exists in healthcare, where doctors reputedly reign supreme and everyone else cowers in fear and scurries around like mice doing their bidding. I had to grudgingly admit that he was absolutely right.

It goes without saying that this dictatorship-like approach to healthcare is extremely outdated and could not be further from the truth in modern healthcare. It is widely recognised that each profession brings their own set of skills and knowledge to the table. Doctors diagnose the condition, pharmacists manage the drugs needed, and nurses administer the drugs and closely monitor the patient. Occupational therapists help the patient carry on with their daily activities, speech pathologists deal with swallowing issues, and dieticians devise a specialised diet according to a patient's requirements. The list goes on. The key to achieving the highest standard of patient care is to put these people in the same room and get them working together. If one leg is removed, the table collapses.

However, societal perceptions are considerably more difficult to change. Perceptions amongst the public, and occasionally within the healthcare industry itself.

It's a bitter pill to swallow, but there are valid reasons as to why these perceptions are so deeply rooted in society. Take a doctor and a pharmacist. The doctor diagnoses a case of community-acquired pneumonia, and the pharmacist recommends the best antibiotic choice and dosing regimen for the individual based on their unique characteristics.

Most of the time, this is not what the public sees. They see the doctor diagnosing a case of community-acquired pneumonia. They see the pharmacist pick the right medicines off the shelf according to the doctor's prescription, stick some labels on and package them in a little doggy bag.

However, what they don't see is the pharmacist checking the literature and the patient's electronic patient record to determine the most appropriate dosing regimen for them, or whether the prescribed antibiotics are the best choice in the first place. The pharmacist evaluates whether the patient's renal and hepatic function is capable of handling the recommended dosing, or if there are any other factors that need to be taken into account. If they happen to be allergic to the antibiotics recommended, the pharmacist sources a safe alternative and justifies this decision with a scientific rationale. The pharmacist checks if the patient has other comorbidities and corresponding medicines to manage. If there is an interaction with a pre-existing condition or medicine, the pharmacist evaluates whether this interaction can be managed safely or if it should be avoided altogether.

The public does not see any of this.

What they do see is the pharmacist staring at the computer screen for a while, maybe looking slightly brain-dead depending on how sleep deprived they are. They see the pharmacist get the right drug off the shelf, count some pills and stick a label on the box.

The most fundamental parts of the profession are the least visible to the public eye. I find this both fascinating and alarming in equal measure.

Occasionally, some healthcare professionals buy into these perceptions themselves. When a patient asks a pharmacist why they take so long to stick a label on a box, the pharmacist may go home that night feeling a little disappointed and undervalued. Over time, the pharmacist may start to believe that labelling boxes is the most significant part of their job. They don't even bother to justify the importance of their clinical work anymore. If all these patients are picking on the same thing, there must be some truth in it – right?

Someday, my friend will ace his prescribing qualification and give these pharmacists the shot of ego boosting juice they desperately need. Maybe an intramuscular one for a longer duration of action.

Remember those folks I mentioned at the very beginning, who asked "Why don't you just become a doctor instead?" Well, here's my answer.

There are far too many things I enjoy about Pharmacy that I may not have discovered had I gone into medicine. I love pharmaceutical science and learning about the principles of drug formulation. I learned that the physicochemical properties of a drug can influence the design of its manufacturing process – and in turn, the nature of the manufacturing process can influence the resulting pharmacokinetic profile. This fascinates me to no end. In the clinical arena, I love that an understanding of pharmacokinetics helps clinical pharmacists spot medication problems that may have gone unnoticed by the rest of the healthcare team. As for cutting edge developments, inhaled drug delivery is an area that holds so much promise, particularly in the midst of the current era of biologics and gene therapy. I am so lucky to have had the opportunity to explore it first-hand as part of my university research project.

Sadly, I don't usually get a chance to fly the pharmacy flag before someone pipes up asking how much money a pharmacist makes.

Acknowledgements

This is for all the weird and wonderful souls whom I have had the pleasure of meeting at some point during my Pharmacy journey. Thank you for all your support, tough love and for inspiring me to write this book. Duncan, thank you for being a wonderful tutor and believing in me when I had no idea what I was doing. To all my professors and lecturers, you taught me everything I know – and made me realise just how much I don't know. Special thanks to Stephen Fletcher in Pharmacy Placements for replying every whiny email of mine and even offering to pre-order a copy of this book.

To my parents, for creating me and constantly worrying about me ever since.

To David, for putting up with me over the past two years – I think that says it all.

Last but certainly not least, thank you to the pond frogs, the goldfish and the neighbour's cat for keeping me company in the garden whilst I wrote this.

References

1.   Khedraki, R., Noor, Z., & Rick, J. (2016). The Most Expensive Drug in the World: To Continue or Discontinue, That Is the Question. *Federal Practitioner : For the Health Care Professionals of the VA, DoD, and PHS, 33*(7), 22–28.

2.   Hughes, J. P., Rees, S. S., Kalindjian, S. B., & Philpott, K. L. (2011, March). Principles of early drug discovery. *British Journal of Pharmacology*, Vol. 162, pp. 1239–1249. https://doi.org/10.1111/j.1476-5381.2010.01127.x

3.   Lal, & Renu. (2015). Patents and Exclusivity. *FDA/CDER Small Business and Industry Assistance Team (SBIA) Chronicles.*

4.   World Health Organisation (2002). *The IMPORTANCE of PHARMACOVIGILANCE Safety Monitoring of medicinal products.*

5.   National Institute of Medical Herbalists. Herbalism. Accessed 01 June 2020, from https://nimh.org.uk/herbalism/

6.   Novković, V. M., Stanojević, L. P., Cakić, M. D., Palić, R. M., Veljković, V. B., & Stanković, M. Z. (2014). Extraction of Digoxin from Fermented Woolly Foxglove Foliage by Percolation. *Separation*

Science and Technology (Philadelphia), *49*(6), 829–837.
https://doi.org/10.1080/01496395.2013.864679

7.   Royal Pharmaceutical Society. The Traditional Herbal Medicine Registration Scheme - Quick reference guide. Accessed 01 June 2020, from https://www.rpharms.com/resources/quick-reference-guides/herbal-medicine-registration-scheme-2

8.   Directive 2004/24/EC of the European Parliament and of the Council. (2004). *Official Journal of the European Union*. Accessed 01 June 2020, from
https://ec.europa.eu/health/sites/health/files/files/eudralex/vol-1/dir_2004_24/dir_2004_24_en.pdf

9.   Welcome to the GRCCT. Accessed 01 June 2020, from The General Regulatory Council for Complementary Therapies website: http://www.grcct.org/about-us/

10.   Joint Formulary Committee. *British National Formulary* (online) London: BMJ Group and Pharmaceutical Press. Accessed on 01 June 2020, from http://www.medicinescomplete.com

11.   Hildebrandt, A. G. (2004). Pharmacology, drug efficacy, and the individual. *Drug Metabolism Reviews*, Vol. 36, pp. 845–852. https://doi.org/10.1081/DMR-200033500

12.   Directive 2010/63/EU of the European Parliament and of the Council of 22 September 2010 on the protection of animals used for scientific purposes. Accessed 08 June 2020, from https://eur-lex.europa.eu/legal-content/EN/TXT/?uri=celex%3A32010L0063

13. nhs.uk. Exercise – Physical activity guidelines for adults aged 19 to 64. Accessed 24 June 2020, from https://www.nhs.uk/live-well/exercise/

About the Author

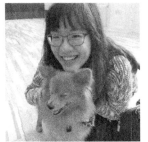 Janelle Soong was born in Malaysia and emigrated to England at the age of ten on a music scholarship. She graduated from King's College London in 2020 with First Class Honours in Pharmacy (MPharm).

Let Sleeping Pharmacists Lie is her first book, inspired by her personal encounters as a Pharmacy student. She also draws on her work experience within the retail, hospital and industrial sectors.

Janelle manages and writes regularly for her blog (thenellybean.com). This serves as a creative outlet where she posts opinionated rants, pieces on funny daily observations and anything else that takes her fancy.

Outside work, Janelle can usually be found enjoying a Tchaikovsky symphony with a cup of tea, whilst planning her next baking project – usually involving chocolate in some shape or form.

 twitter.com/thenellybean

 instagram.com/janelle_thenellybean